The Complete Plant-Based Meal Cooking Guide

A Collection of Plant-Based Lunch and Dinner Recipes to Start Your Diet and Boost Your Days

Sheryl Ward

Table of Contents

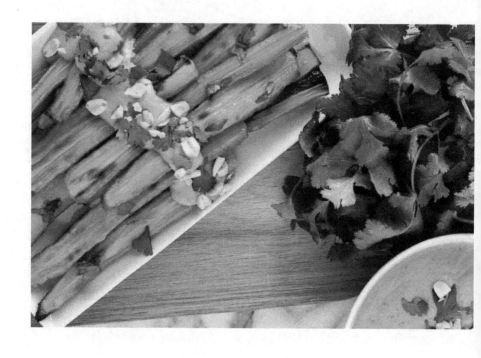

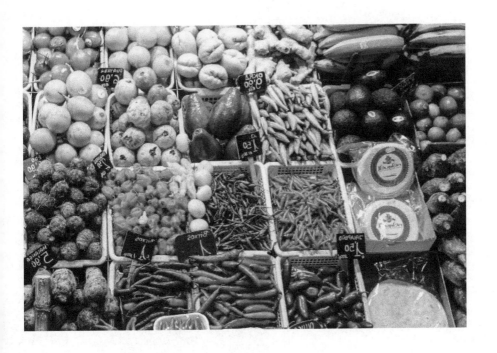

Cauliflower Mash

Preparation time: 10 minutesCooking time: 10 minutes
Servings: 4

Ingredients:

1 head of cauliflower ¼ tsp, garlic powder 1 handful of chives, chopped What you'll need from the store cupboard: ¼ tsp, salt ¼ tsp, ground black pepper

Directions

Bring a pot of water to boil. Chop cauliflower into florets. Place in a pot of boiling water and boil for 5 minutes. Drain well. Place florets in a blender. Add remaining ingredients except for chives and pulse to desired consistency. Transfer to a bowl and toss in chives. Serve and enjoy.

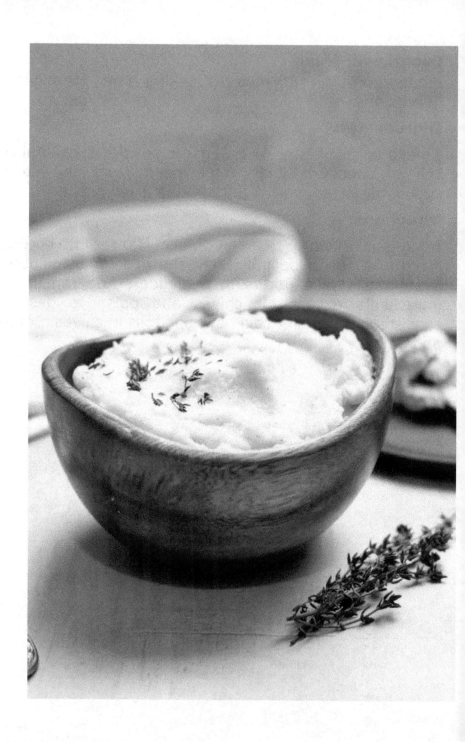

Keto Enchilada Bake

Preparation time: 10 minutesCooking time: 20 minutes
Servings: 6

Ingredients:

1 package House Foods Organic Extra Firm Tofu 1 cup roma tomatoes, chopped 1 cup shredded cheddar cheese 1 small avocado, pitted and sliced ½ cup sour cream What you'll need from the store cupboard: 5 tablespoons olive oil Salt and pepper to taste

Directions

Preheat oven to 3500F. Cut tofu into small cubes and sauté with oil and seasoning. Set aside and reserve the oil. Place the tofu in the bottom of a casserole dish. Mix the reserved oil and tomatoes and pour over the tofu. Sprinkle with cheese on top. Bake for 20 minutes. Top with avocado and sour cream toppings. Serve and enjoy.

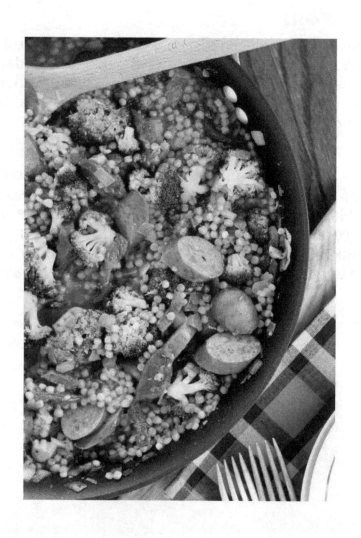

Creamy Kale and Mushrooms

Preparation time: 10 minutes Cooking time: 15 minutes Servings: 3

Ingredients:

3 cloves of garlic, minced 1 onion, chopped 1 bunch kale, stems removed and leaves chopped 3 white button mushrooms, chopped 1 cup heavy cream What you'll need from the store cupboard: 5 tablespoons oil Salt and pepper to taste

Directions

Heat oil in a pot. Sauté the garlic and onion until fragrant for 2 minutes. Stir in mushrooms. Season with pepper and salt. Cook for 8 minutes. Stir in kale and coconut milk. Simmer for 5 minutes. Adjust seasoning to taste.

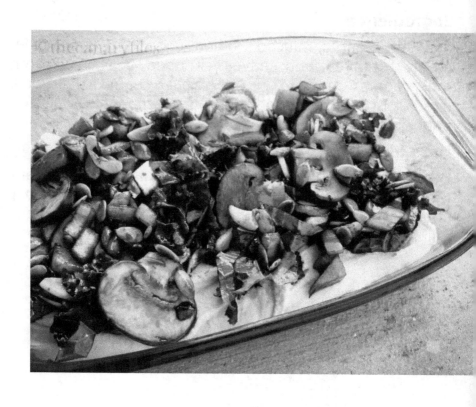

Stir Fried Bok Choy

Preparation time: minutesCooking time: 15 minutes Servings: 4

Ingredients:

4 cloves of garlic, minced 1 onion, chopped 2 heads bok choy, rinsed and chopped 2 tablespoons sesame oil 2 tablespoons sesame seeds, toasted What you'll need from the store cupboard: 3 tablespoons oil Salt and pepper to taste

Directions

Heat the oil in a pot for 2 minutes. Sauté the garlic and onions until fragrant, around 3 minutes. Stir in the bok choy, salt, and pepper. Cover pan and cook for 5 minutes. Stir and continue cooking for another 3 minutes. Drizzle with sesame oil and sesame seeds on top before serving.

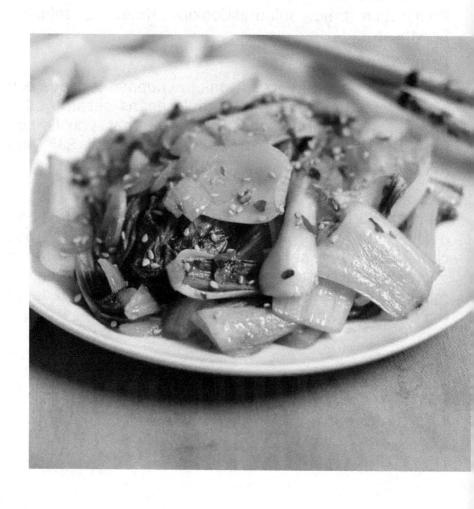

Sweet and Sour Tofu

Ingredients:

½ tablespoon coconut oil 1 firm tofu, sliced into strips 1 onion, chopped 1 garlic clove, minced 1 red pepper, chopped 1 green pepper, chopped 1 cup brown rice, cooked

For the Sauce:

3 tablespoon brown rice vinegar 2 tablespoons tomato paste ½ tablespoon tamari ½ tablespoon water ½ tablespoon corn starch

Directions:

In a small bowl, combine cornstarch and water. Set aside. Meanwhile, in a saucepan, put together tomato paste, and vinegar. Allow to simmer for 10 minutes. Add in cornstarch. Stir well until the sauce thickens. Meanwhile, preheat the broiler. Prepare a baking pan lined with baking sheet. Dip tofu in the sauce. Line in a baking sheet. Broil for 5 minutes, flip to make sure all sides are coated well. Continue broiling for 5 more minutes. In a pan, pour coconut oil. Saute onion, garlic, and bell pepper for 3 minutes or until softened. Set aside. Serve by placing broiled tofu on top of bed of greens or rice. Pt sautéed veggies on the side.

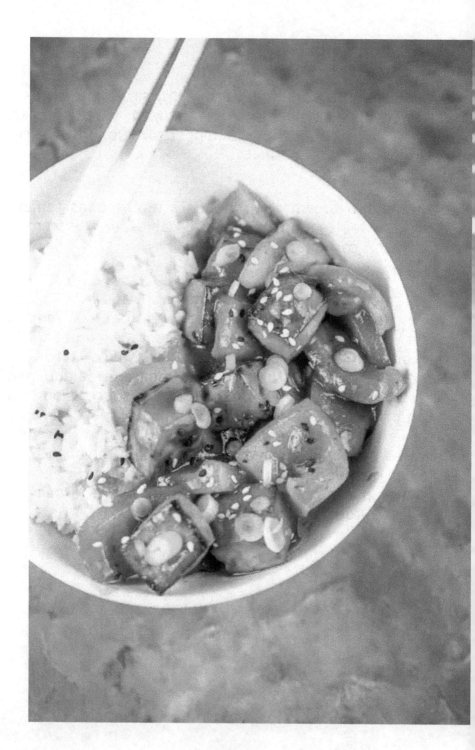

Grilled Parmesan Eggplant

Preparation time: 5 minutesCooking time: 15 minutes
Servings: 4

Ingredients:

1 medium-sized eggplant 1 log (1 pound) fresh mozzarella cheese, cut into sixteen slices 1 small tomato, cut into eight slices 1/2 cup shredded Parmesan cheese Chopped fresh basil or parsley What you'll need from the store cupboard: 1/2 teaspoon salt 1 tablespoon olive oil 1/2 teaspoon pepper

Directions

Trim ends of the eggplant; cut eggplant crosswise into eight slices. Sprinkle with salt; let stand 5 minutes. Blot eggplant dry with paper towels; brush both sides with oil and sprinkle with pepper. Grill, covered, over medium heat 4-6 minutes on each side or until tender. Remove from grill. Top eggplant with mozzarella cheese, tomato, and Parmesan cheese. Grill, covered, 1-2 minutes longer or until cheese begins to melt. Top with basil.

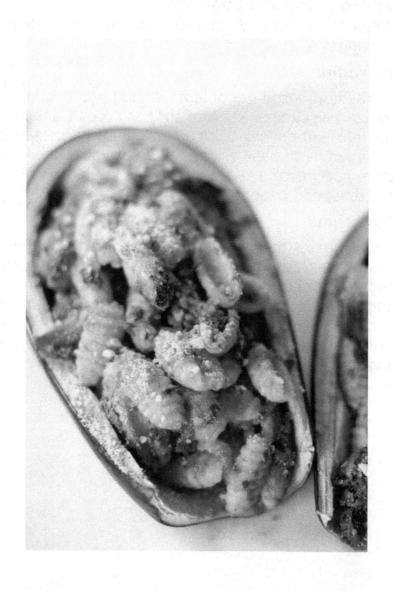

Curried Tofu

Preparation time: 5 minutesCooking time: 15 minutes
Servings: 6

Ingredients:

2 cloves of garlic, minced 1 onion, cubed 12-ounce firm tofu, drained and cubed 1 teaspoon curry powder 1 tablespoon soy sauce What you'll need from the store cupboard: ¼ teaspoon pepper 5 tablespoons olive oil

Directions

Heat the oil in a skillet over medium flame. Sauté the garlic and onion until fragrant. Stir in the tofu and stir for 3 minutes. Add the rest of the ingredients and adjust the water. Close the lid and allow simmering for 10 minutes. Serve and enjoy.

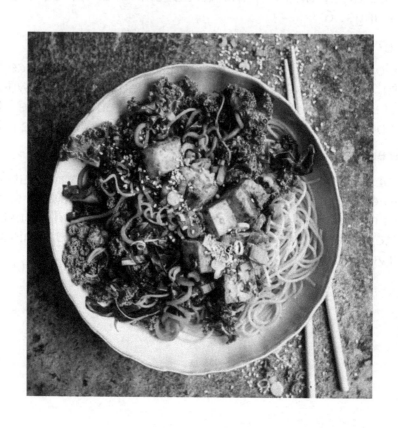

Lemon Garlic Broccoli

Preparation Time: 10 minutes Cooking Time: 10 minutes Servings: 2

Ingredients:

2 teaspoons olive oil 3 cloves garlic, minced 2 cups broccoli, sliced into florets Salt and pepper to taste 1 tablespoon freshly squeezed lemon juice

Direction

In a pan over medium heat, pour the olive oil. Once hot, add the garlic and cook for 30 seconds. Add the broccoli florets and cook until tender Stir in the lemon juice. Let cool. Put in a food container and reheat when ready to eat.

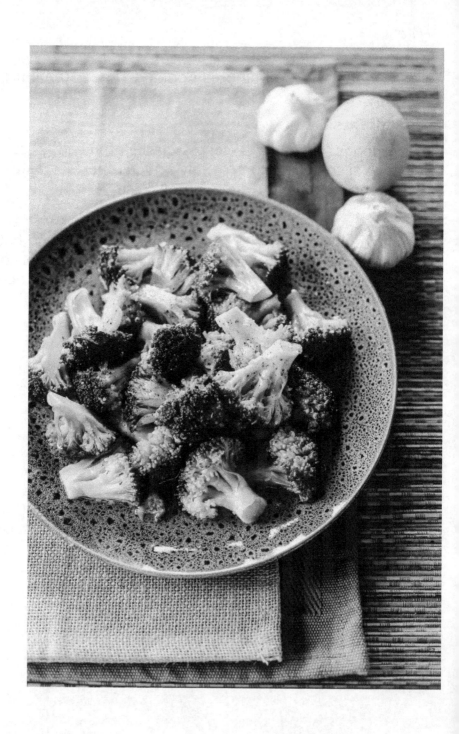

Collard Greens with Shiitake Mushrooms

Preparation Time: 15 minutes Cooking Time: 10 minutes Servings: 4

Ingredients:

¼ teaspoon salt ¾ teaspoon smoked paprika ¼ teaspoon red pepper, crushed ¼ teaspoon ground cumin ¾ cup reduced-sodium vegetable broth 2 tablespoons olive oil 4 cloves garlic, minced 5 oz. shiitake mushrooms, chopped 16 oz. collard greens, chopped 2 tablespoons cider vinegar 1 teaspoon hot sauce ½ teaspoon ground pepper

Direction

Add salt, paprika, red pepper, cumin and broth in a pan over medium heat. Simmer for 1 minute, stirring to blend well. Transfer to a plate and set aside. In a pot over medium high heat, add the oil. Cook the garlic and mushrooms for 4 minutes. Pour 2 tablespoons of the paprika mixture to the pot. Mix well. Add the collard greens and gradually add the remaining paprika mixture. Stir in the rest of the Ingredients. Cook for 1 minute. Store in a food container and reheat when ready to eat.

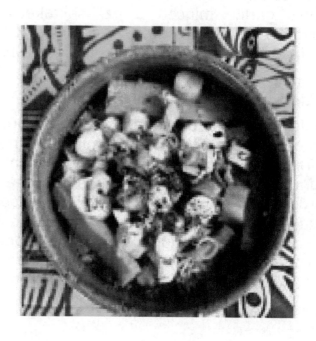

Mashed Potato with Carrots & Corn

Preparation Time: 15 minutes Cooking Time: 30 minutes
Servings: 4

Ingredients:

Water 8 potatoes, peeled and cubed Salt 4 tablespoons
vegan butter, divided 1 cup frozen corn and carrot cubes
Salt and pepper to taste 1 cup pecans 2 tablespoons
flaxseeds

Direction

Fill a pot with water. Put in the stove and bring to a boil.
Add the potatoes. Simmer until the potatoes are tender.
Take the potatoes out of the pot and drain. Mash the
potatoes using a fork or a masher. Stir in 3 tablespoons
butter. Season with salt and pepper. In a pan over
medium heat, add remaining butter. Add the frozen
vegetables. Sauté for 3 minutes. Drain the liquid. Divide
the mashed potato in food containers. Top with the cubed
corn and carrots. Reheat before serving.

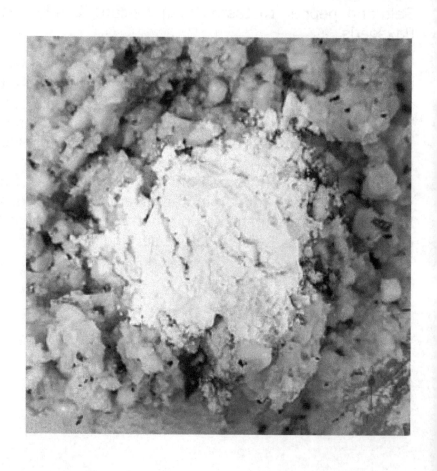

Glazed Carrots

Preparation Time: 10 minutes Cooking time: 4 hours Servings: 10

Ingredients:

1 pound parsnips, cut into medium chunks 2 pounds carrots, cut into medium chunks 2 tablespoons orange peel, shredded 1 cup orange juice ½ cup orange marmalade ½ cup veggie stock 1 tablespoon tapioca, crushed A pinch of salt and black pepper 3 tablespoons olive oil ¼ cup parsley, chopped

Directions:

In your slow cooker, mix parsnips with carrots. In a bowl, mix orange peel with orange juice, stock, orange marmalade, tapioca, salt and pepper, whisk and add over carrots. Cover slow cooker and cook everything on High for 4 hours. Add parsley, toss, divide between plates and serve as a side dish. Enjoy!

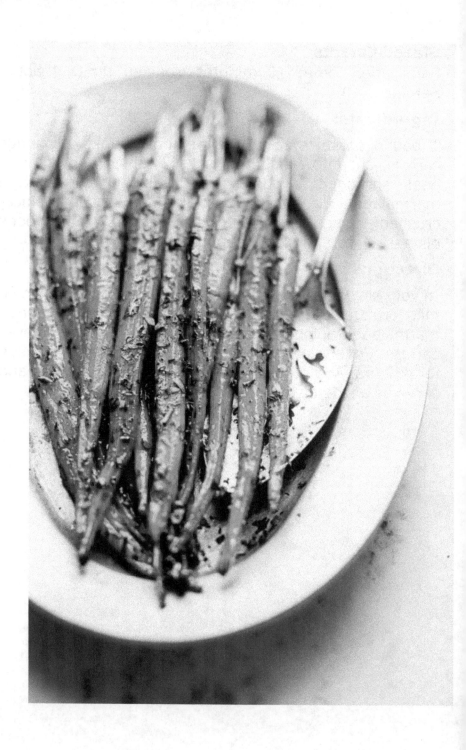

Squash And Spinach Mix

Preparation Time: 10 minutes Cooking time: 3 hours and 30 minutes Servings: 12

Ingredients:

10 ounces spinach, torn 2 pounds butternut squash, peeled and cubed 1 cup barley 1 yellow onion, chopped 14 ounces veggie stock ½ cup water A pinch of salt and black pepper to the taste 3 garlic cloves, minced

Directions:

In your slow cooker, mix squash with spinach, barley, onion, stock, water, salt, pepper and garlic, toss, cover and cook on High for 3 hours and 30 minutes. Divide squash mix on plates and serve as a side dish. Enjoy!

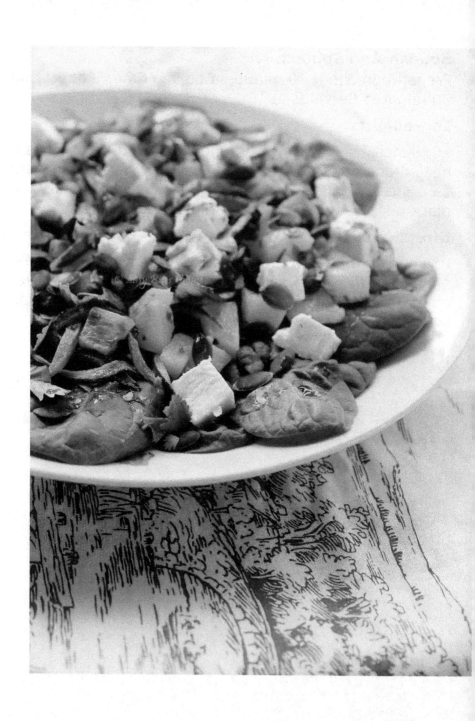

Cream of Carrot and Potato Soup

Preparation time: 5 minutes Cooking time: 50 minutes
Servings: 3

Ingredients:

3 cups carrots, sliced 2 potatoes, diced 1 yellow onion, chopped 4 Tbs. flour ½ cup olive oil 1 tsp. sugar ½ cup water 1½ cups light cream 4½ cups milk paprika cayenne pepper 1 clove garlic, minced (optional) brandy garnish 1 tsp. salt fresh-ground black pepper chopped parsley, for garnish

Directions:

Sauté the carrots and onions in a large skillet or soup pot in 4 tablespoons of olive oil for a few minutes. Add the sugar, 1 tsp. salt, the diced potato, and the water. Cover tightly and simmer until the vegetables are just tender. Purée the vegetables in a blender with the cream. Melt the remaining 4 tablespoons butter in a skillet and stir in the flour. Cook the roux until it is golden. Heat the milk and stir it into the roux with a whisk. Cook the white sauce over a very small flame, stirring often, until it is thickened. Combine the carrot purée and the white sauce in a large pot. Grate in some pepper and add paprika and cayenne to taste, as well as a little minced garlic if you like. Add a little brandy and salt to taste. Simmer the soup gently for another 10 or 15 minutes, stirring occasionally. Serve hot, garnished with chopped parsley.

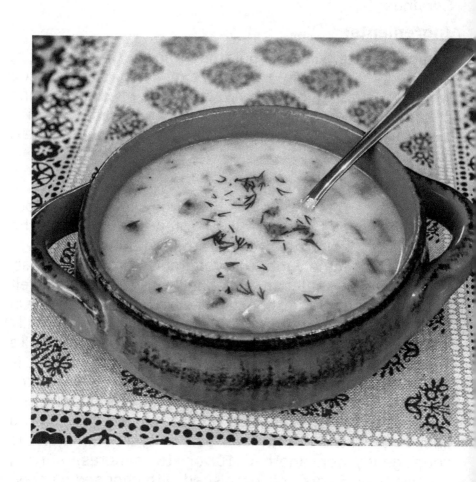

Chilled Tomato Soup

Preparation time: 5 minutes Cooking time: 50 minutes
Servings: 3

Ingredients:

6 tomatoes, medium-sized 1 cucumber, chopped ½ cup
onion, chopped finely 4 tsp. lemon juice 1 Tbs. lemon
rind, grated 1 cup sour cream ½ tsp. ginger 1 large
cantaloupe 1 Tbs. dried basil, crushed 2½ tsp. salt
pepper to taste

Directions:

Put the tomatoes in boiling water for a few minutes, until
the skins start to crack and peel. Remove the tomatoes
and peel them. Purée them in a blender or food processor
at high speed. You should have 5 cups of the fresh
tomato purée. Purée the cucumber and onions in a
blender or food processor and add this to the tomatoes.
If you are using a blender, you could "prime" it with a
bit of the puréed tomatoes. Stir in the sour cream and
season the soup with salt, ginger, pepper, lemon juice,
and lemon rind. Halve the cantaloupe, remove all the
seeds, and either cut it into small balls with a melon
scoop or peel and cut it into chunks. Toss the melon with
the chopped basil and chill both soup and melon for
several hours. To serve, pour the soup into chilled bowls
and put a few spoonful of the melon into each one.

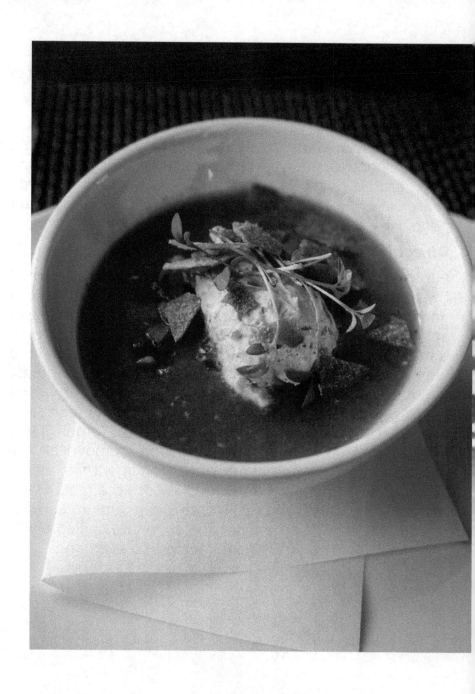

Burst Your Belly Vegan Tortilla Soup

Preparation time: 5 minutes Cooking time: 40 minutes 6 Servings.

Ingredients:

3 minced garlic cloves 1 tbsp. olive oil 1 diced onion ¾ cup quinoa 1 diced green pepper 32 ounces vegetable broth 1 diced zucchini 6 corn tortillas 1 16 ounce can of diced tomatoes 1 tsp. cumin ½ tsp. oregano salt and pepper to taste

Directions:

Begin by heating the oil in a soup pan, and adding the garlic and the onion to the oil. Cook these for five minutes. Afterwards, add the quinoa, the broth, and the bell pepper. Bring this mixture to a boil. Afterwards, lower the heat and allow it to simmer for fifteen minutes. Next, slice up the tortillas into small strips and heat them in a skillet with a little olive oil in order to toast them. Now, add the zucchini, the cumin, and the oregano to the soup. Stir, and allow it to simmer for fifteen more minutes. Add salt and pepper, and serve warm with tortilla strips overtop. Enjoy!

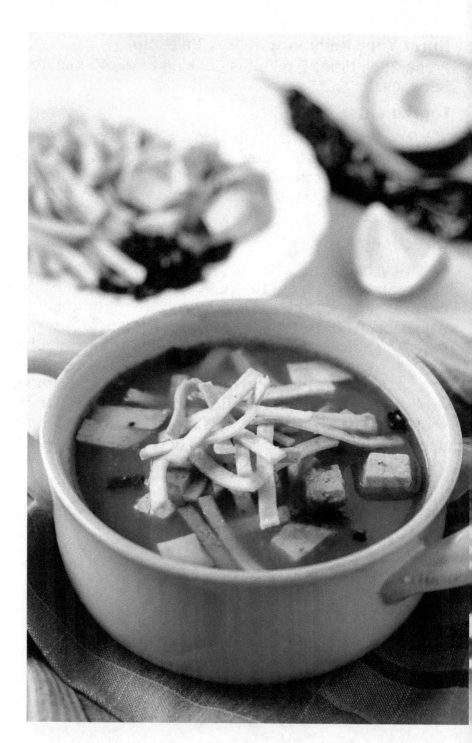

Protein-Revving Lentil Vegetable Soup

Preparation time: 5 minutes Cooking time: 50 minutes 8 Servings.

Ingredients:

3 minced garlic cloves 1 diced onion 3 tbsp. olive oil 2 sliced carrots 2 diced celery stalks 5 cups water 2 diced potatoes 1 tbsp. Italian herbs 1 ½ cups green lentils 2 tsp. paprika 16 ounces diced tomatoes 1/3 cup chopped cilantro

Directions:

Begin by heating the oil and the vegetables together in the bottom of a soup pot. Saute the vegetables for about ten minutes. Afterwards, add the water, the lentils, the potatoes, the seasoning, and the paprika. Stir, and allow the mixture to simmer for thirty minutes with the cover on. Next, place the cilantro in the soup and allow it to simmer for twenty more minutes. Serve with a bit of salt and pepper, and enjoy.

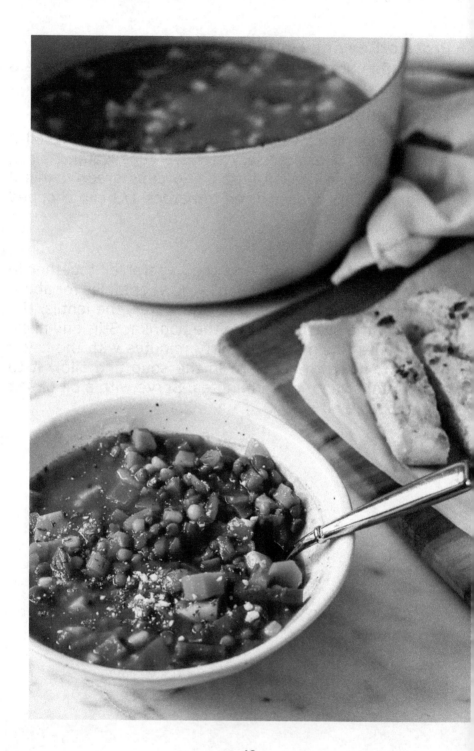

Kimchi Pasta

Preparation time: 5 minutes Cooking time: 25 minutes Servings: 4

Ingredients:

2 1/3 Cup Vegetable Stock 8 Ounces Small Pasta 2 Cloves Garlic, Minced ½ Red Onion, Sliced 1 Teaspoon Sea Salt, Fine 1 ¼ Cups Kimchi, Chopped ½ Cup Cashew Sour Cream

Directions:

Combine the stock, garlic, red onion, pasta and salt in your instant pot. Lock the lid, and cook on high pressure for a minute. Use a quick release, and then press sauté and set it to low. Stir the kimchi in, and allow it to simmer for three minutes. Stir in the sour cream before serving warm.

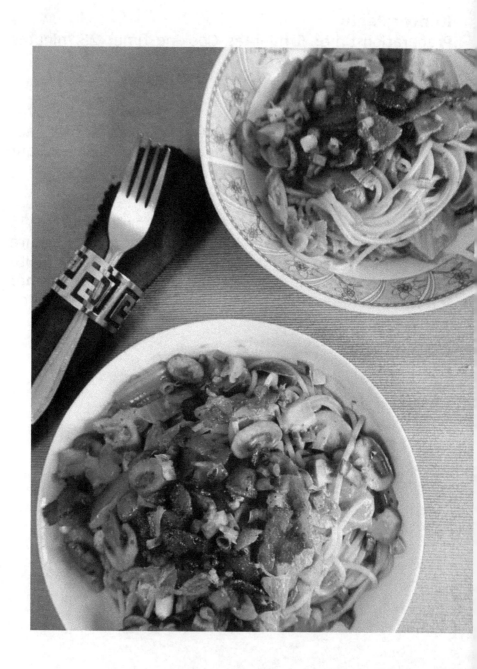

Garlic Lemon Mushrooms

Preparation time: 15 minutesCooking time: 20 minutes
Servings: 4

Ingredients:

1/4 cup lemon juice 3 tablespoons minced fresh parsley 3 garlic cloves, minced 1-pound large fresh mushrooms What you'll need from the store cupboard: Pepper to taste 4 tablespoons olive oil

Directions

For the dressing, whisk together the first 5 ingredients. Toss mushrooms with 2 tablespoons dressing. Grill mushrooms, covered, over medium-high heat until tender, 5-7 minutes per side. Toss with remaining dressing before serving.

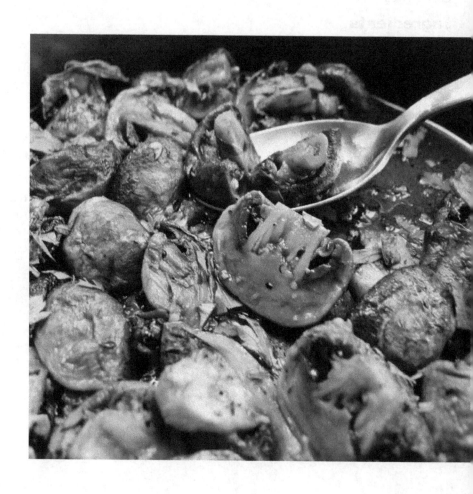

Grilled Spicy Eggplant

Preparation time: 20 minutesCooking time: 20 minutes
Servings: 2

Ingredients:

2 small eggplants, cut into 1/2-inch slices 1/4 cup olive oil 2 tablespoons lime juice 3 teaspoons Cajun seasoning What you'll need from the store cupboard: Salt and pepper to taste

Directions:

Brush eggplant slices with oil. Drizzle with lime juice; sprinkle with Cajun seasoning. Let stand for 5 minutes. Grill eggplant, covered, over medium heat or broil 4 minutes. from heat until tender, 4-5 minutes per side. Season with pepper and salt to taste. Serve and enjoy.

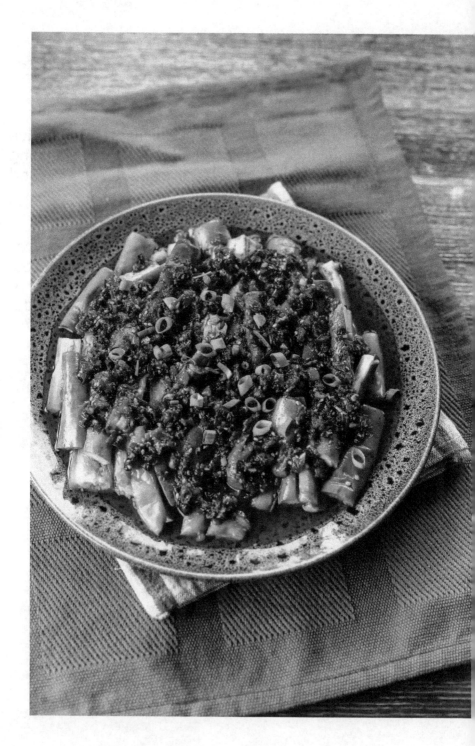

Zucchini Garlic Fries

Preparation time: minutesCooking time: 25 minutes Servings: 6

Ingredients:

¼ teaspoon garlic powder ½ cup almond flour 2 large egg, beaten 3 medium zucchinis, sliced into fry sticks 3 tablespoons olive oil What you'll need from the store cupboard: Salt and pepper to taste

Directions

Preheat oven to 400oF. Mix all ingredients in a bowl until the zucchini fries are well coated. Place fries on a cookie sheet and spread evenly. Put in the oven and cook for 15 minutes. Stir fries, continue baking for an additional 10 minutes.

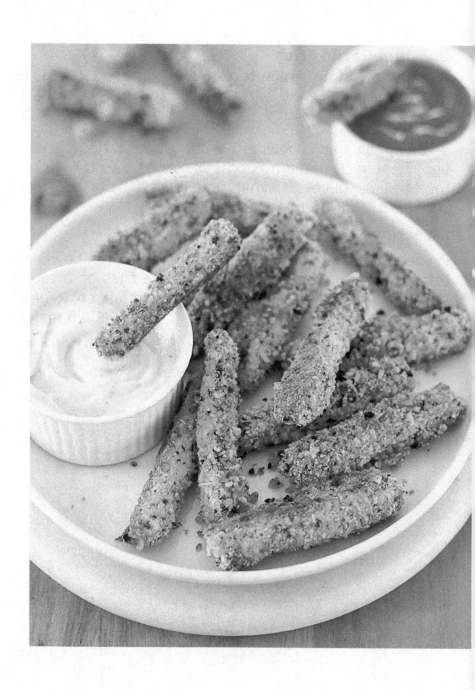

Provolone Over Herbed Portobello Mushrooms

Preparation time: 10 minutesCooking time: 10 minutes
Servings: 2

Ingredients:

2 Portobello mushrooms, stemmed and wiped clean 1 tsp minced garlic ¼ tsp dried rosemary 1 tablespoon balsamic vinegar ¼ cup grated provolone cheese What you'll need from the store cupboard: 4 tablespoons olive oil Salt and pepper to taste

Directions

In an oven, position rack 4-inches away from the top and preheat broiler. Prepare a baking dish by spraying with cooking spray lightly. Stemless, place mushroom gill side up. Mix well garlic, rosemary, balsamic vinegar, and olive oil in a small bowl. Season with salt and pepper to taste. Drizzle over mushrooms equally. Marinate for at least 5 minutes before popping into the oven and broiling for 4 minutes per side or until tender. Once cooked, remove from oven, sprinkle cheese, return to broiler and broil for a minute or two or until cheese melts. Remove from oven and serve right away.

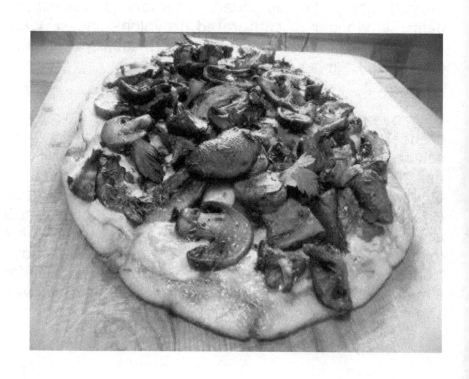

Blue Cheese, Fig and Arugula Salad

Preparation time: 10 minutesCooking time: 0 minutes Servings: 4

Ingredients:

1 tsp Dijon mustard 3 tbsp Balsamic Vinegar ¼ cup crumbled blue cheese 2 bags arugula 1 fig fruit, sliced ½ cup walnuts, chopped What you'll need from the store cupboard: Pepper and salt to taste 5 tbsp olive oil

Directions

Whisk thoroughly together pepper, salt, olive oil, Dijon mustard, and balsamic vinegar to make the dressing. Set aside in the ref for at least 30 minutes to marinate and allow the spices to combine. On four serving plates, evenly arrange arugula and top with blue cheese, figs, and walnuts Drizzle each plate of salad with 1 ½ tbsp of prepared dressing. Serve and enjoy.

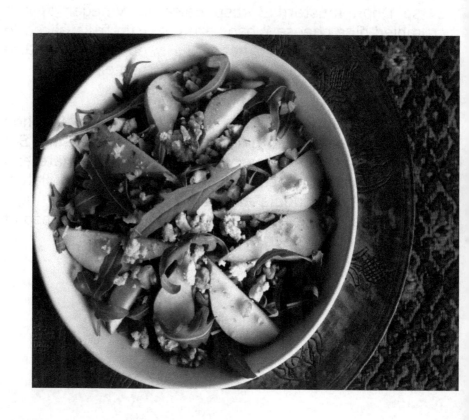

Paprika 'n Cajun Seasoned Onion Rings

Preparation time: 15 minutesCooking time: 25 minutes
Servings: 6

Ingredients:

1 large white onion 2 large eggs, beaten ½ teaspoon Cajun seasoning ¾ cup almond flour 1 ½ teaspoon paprika What you'll need from the store cupboard: ½ cups coconut oil for frying ¼ cup water Salt and pepper to taste

Directions

Preheat a pot with oil for 8 minutes. Peel the onion, cut off the top and slice into circles. In a mixing bowl, combine the water and the eggs. Season with pepper and salt. Soak the onion in the egg mixture. In another bowl, combine the almond flour, paprika powder, Cajun seasoning, salt and pepper. Dredge the onion in the almond flour mixture. Place in the pot and cook in batches until golden brown, around 8 minutes per batch.

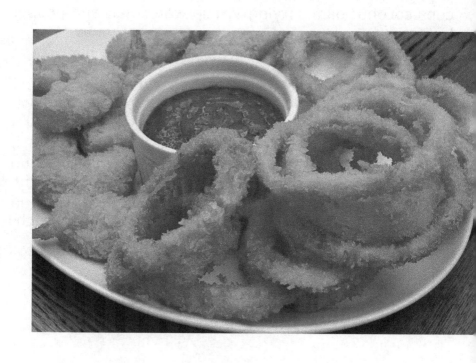

Vegetable Soup

Preparation time: 5 minutes Cooking time: 40 minutes Servings: 6

Ingredients:

12 Ounces Green Beans 1 Can Tomatoes, Diced 1 Onion, Chopped 12 Ounces Mixed Vegetables, Frozen 2 ¾ Cup Vegetable Broth

Directions:

Press sauté, and then add in some cooking oil. Add the onion, and sauté for two minutes. Stir in the remaining ingredients. Seal the lid, and then cook on high pressure for five minutes. Use a natural release for five minutes before finishing with a quick release. Serve warm.

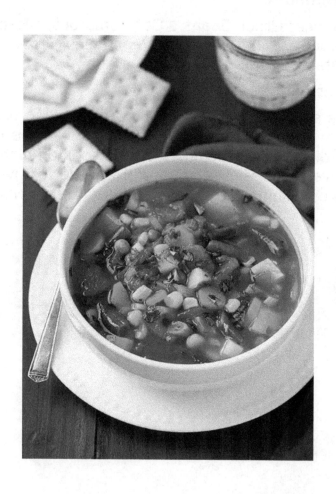

Spinach & Tomato Couscous

Preparation time: 5 minutes Cooking time: 35 minutes Servings: 4

Ingredients:

1 ¼ Vegetable Broth 8 Ounces Couscous 1 ½ Cups Tomatoes, Chopped 2 Tablespoons Vegan Butter ½ Cup Spinach, Fresh & Chopped

Directions:

Press sauté on your instant pot, and melt your butter. Once the butter I smelted, stir in the couscous, allowing it to cook for a minute. Pour in the broth, and stir well before sealing the lid. Cook on high pressure for five minutes, and then use a quick release. Stir in your tomato and spinach, and serve warm.

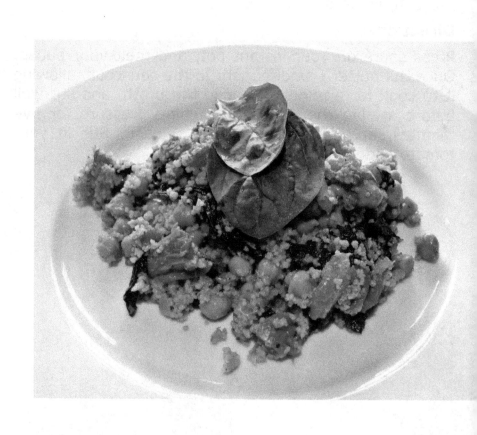

Basil Risotto

Preparation time: 5 minutes Cooking time: 40 minutes Servings: 6

Ingredients:

1 Onion, Chopped 1 ½ Tablespoons Olive Oil 28 Ounces Vegetable Broth 12 Ounces Arborio Rice 1 ½ Cups Basil, Chopped & Fresh

Directions:

Turn your instant pot on sauté and warm your oil. Chop the onions before adding them. Cook for three minutes, and then add in your rice. Cook for a minute more before adding in your broth. Stir well, and then seal the lid. Cook for fifteen minutes on high pressure. Use a quick release, and then press sauté. Cook for one more minute, and then serve warm.

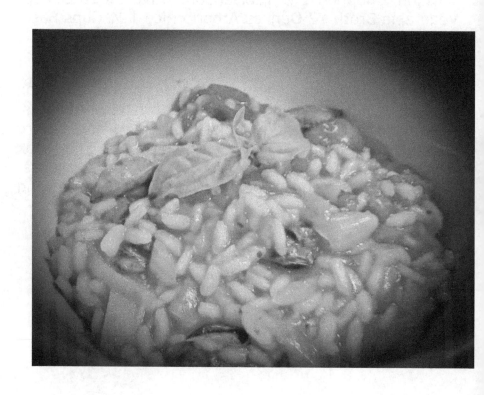

Wild Rice Soup

Preparation time: 5 minutes Cooking time: 20 minutes
Servings: 4

Ingredients:

8 Ounces Baby Bella Mushrooms, Sliced 2 Bay eaves ½
Teaspoon Thyme ½ Teaspoon Paprika 4 Cloves Garlic,
Minced 1 Sweet Onion, Small & Diced 5 Carrots, Sliced 5
Celery Stalks, Sliced 8 Tablespoons Vegan Butter,
Divided ½ Teaspoon Sea Salt 4 Cups Vegetable Stock ½
Cups All Purpose Flour 1 Cup Coconut Milk 1 Cup Wild
Rice Black Pepper to Taste

Directions: Press sauté, and then add in your butter.
Once your butter has melted, add in your celery, carrots,
onion, mushrooms, garlic, paprika, bay leaves, thyme
and salt. Cook for three minutes, and then turn it off of
sauté. Stir in the wild rice and stock. Seal the lid, and
then cook on high pressure for thirty-five minutes. Get
out a small pan and place it over medium-low heat, and
then melt six tablespoons of butter. Whisk in your flour,
allowing it to cook for four minutes. Whisk in the milk,
and make sure to continue whisking until it creates a
lump free mixture. Use a quick release, and the discard
the bay leaves. Press sauté, and then stir in your butter
mixture. Cook until it thickens, and then season with salt
and pepper before serving warm.

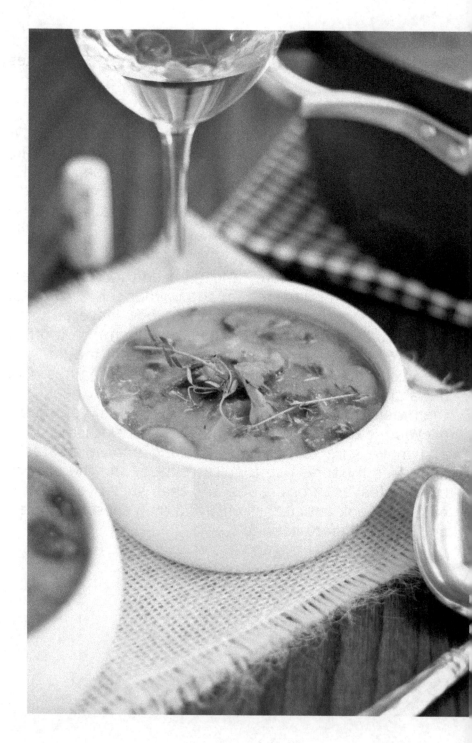

Brussels Sprout and Lentil Soup

Preparation time: 5 minutes Cooking time: 40 minutes
Servings: 4

Ingredients:

1 cup brown lentils 1 onion, chopped 2-3 cloves garlic, peeled 2 medium carrots, chopped 16 oz Brussels sprouts, shredded 4 cups vegetable broth 4 tbsp olive oil 1 ½ tsp paprika 1 tsp summer savory

Directions:

Heat oil in a deep soup pot, add the onion and carrots and sauté until golden. Add in paprika and lentils with vegetable broth. Bring to the boil, lower heat and simmer for 15-20 minutes. Add the Brussels sprouts and the tomato to the soup, together with the garlic and summer savory. Cook for 15 more minutes, add salt to taste and serve.

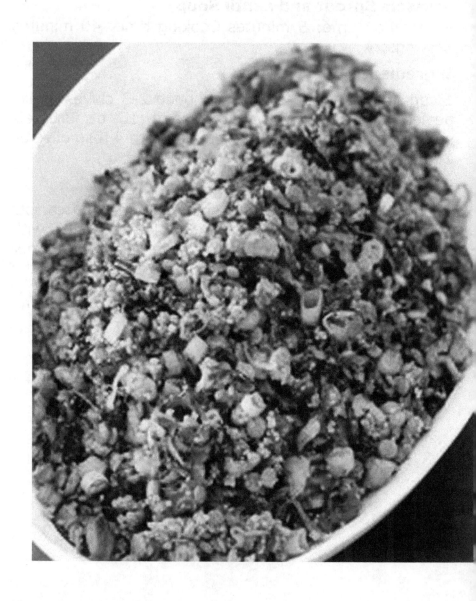

Green Lentil Soup with Rice

Preparation time: 5 minutes Cooking time: 40 minutes
Servings: 6

Ingredients:

1 cup green lentils 1 small onion, finely cut 1 carrot,
chopped 5 cups vegetable broth 1/4 cup rice 1 tbsp
paprika salt and black pepper, to taste 1/2 cup finely cut
dill, to serve

Directions:

Heat oil in a large saucepan and sauté the onion stirring
occasionally, until transparent. Add in carrot, paprika and
lentils and stir to combine. Add vegetable broth to the
saucepan and bring to the boil, then reduce heat and
simmer for 20 minutes. Stir in rice and cook on medium
low until rice is cooked. Sprinkle with dill and serve.

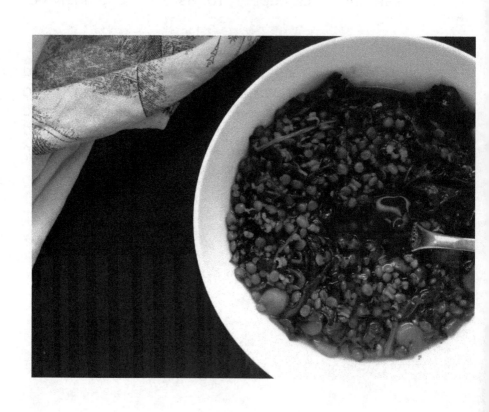

Bean and Pasta Soup

Preparation time: 5 minutes Cooking time: 20 minutes
Servings: 6-7

Ingredients:

1 cup small pasta, cooked 1 cup canned white beans, rinsed and drained 2 medium carrots, cut 1 cup fresh spinach, torn 1 medium onion, chopped 1 celery rib, chopped 2 garlic cloves, crushed 3 cups water 1 cup canned tomatoes, diced and undrained 1 cup vegetable broth ½ tsp rosemary ½ tsp basil salt and pepper, to taste

Directions:

Add all ingredients except pasta and spinach into slow cooker. Cover and cook on low for 6-7 hours or high for 4 hours. Add spinach and pasta about 30 minutes before the soup is finished cooking.

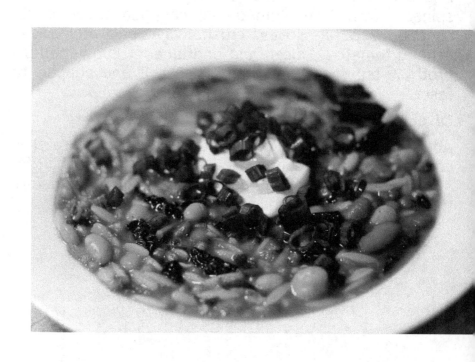

Spiced Citrus Bean Soup

Preparation time: 5 minutes Cooking time: 40 minutes
Servings: 6-7

Ingredients:

1 can (14 oz) white beans, rinsed and drained 2 medium
carrots, cut 1 medium onion, chopped 1 tbsp gram
masala 4 cups vegetable broth 1 cup coconut milk 1/2
tbsp grated ginger juice of 1 orange salt and pepper, to
taste 1/2 cup fresh parsley leaves, finely cut, to serve

Directions:

In a large soup pot, sauté onions, carrots and ginger in
olive oil, for about 5 minutes, stirring. Add gram masala
and cook until just fragrant. Add the orange juice and
vegetable broth and bring to the boil. Simmer for about
10 min until the carrots are tender, then stir in the
coconut milk. Blend soup to desired consistency then add
the beans and bring to a simmer. Serve sprinkled with
parsley.

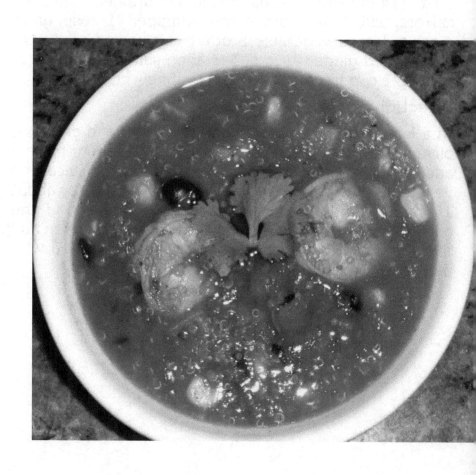

Curried Lentil Squash Stew

Preparation time: 5 minutes Cooking time: 30 minutes 4 Servings.

Ingredients:

1 diced onion 1 tsp. olive oil 4 minced garlic cloves 4 cups vegetable broth 1 tbsp. curry powder 1 cup red lentils 4 cups pre-baked butternut squash 1 cup broccoli

Directions: Begin by bringing the oil, the onion, and the garlic together in the bottom of a soup pot for five minutes on medium. Next, add the curry powder, and stir the ingredients for a few minutes. Add the broth and the lentils to the pot, and allow the mixture to simmer for ten minutes. Next, add the pre-baked butternut squash and the broccoli to the mixture. Allow the soup to cook for ten minutes, stirring occasionally. Add salt, pepper, and curry powder to the mixture to your desired taste, and enjoy.

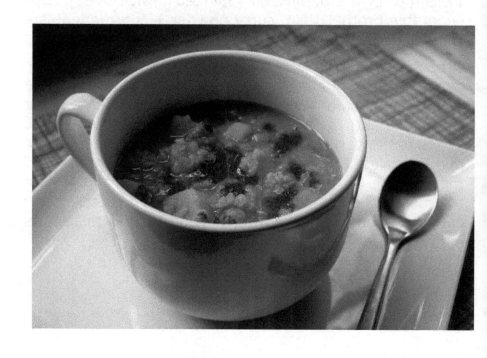

Rich Red Lentil Curry

Servings: 16 Preparation time: 8 hours and 10 minutes

Ingredients:

4 cups of brown lentils, uncooked and rinsed 2 medium-sized white onions, peeled and diced 2 teaspoons of minced garlic 1 tablespoon of minced ginger 1 teaspoon of salt 1/4 teaspoon of cayenne pepper 5 tablespoons of red curry paste 2 teaspoon of brown sugar 1 1/2 teaspoon of ground turmeric 1 tablespoon of garam masala 60-ounce of tomato puree 7 cups of water 1/2 cup of coconut milk 1/4 cup of chopped cilantro

Directions:

Using a 6-quarts slow cooker, place all the ingredients except for the coconut milk and cilantro. Stir until it mixes properly and cover the top. Plug in the slow cooker; adjust the cooking time to 5 hours and let it cook on the high heat setting or until the lentils are soft. Check the curry during cooking and add more water if needed. When the curry is cooked, stir in the milk, then garnish it with the cilantro and serve right away.

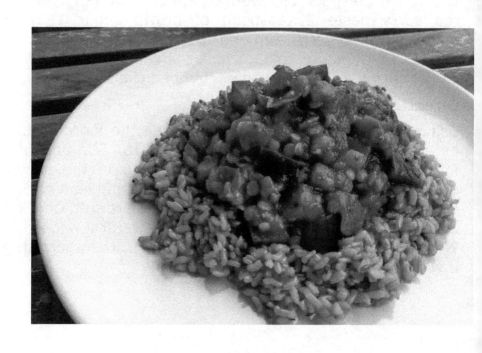

Paprika Broccoli

Preparation Time: 10 minutes Cooking Time: 20 minutes
Servings:

Ingredients

1 broccoli head, florets separated Juice of ½ lemon 1
tablespoon olive oil 2 teaspoons paprika Salt and black
pepper to the taste 3 garlic cloves, minced 1 tablespoon
sesame seeds

Directions:

In a bowl, mix broccoli with lemon juice, oil, paprika, salt,
pepper and garlic and toss to coat. Transfer to your Air
Fryer's basket, cook at 360 ° F for 15 minutes, sprinkle
sesame seeds, cook for 5 minutes more, divide between
plates and serve as a side dish.

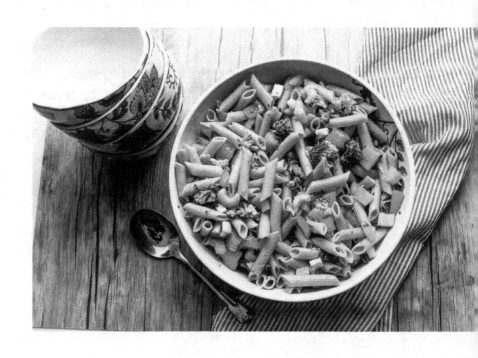

Cajun Onion Mix

Preparation Time: 2 hours Cooking Time: 15 minutes Servings:

Ingredients

2 big white onions, cut into medium chunks Salt and black pepper to the taste ¼ cup coconut cream A drizzle of olive oil 1½ teaspoon paprika 1 teaspoon garlic powder ½ teaspoon Cajun seasoning

Directions:

In a pan that fits your Air Fryer, combine onion chunks with salt, pepper, cream, oil, paprika, garlic powder and Cajun seasoning, toss, introduce the pan in your Air Fryer and cook at 360 ° F for 15 minutes. Divide the onion mix between plates and serve as a side dish.

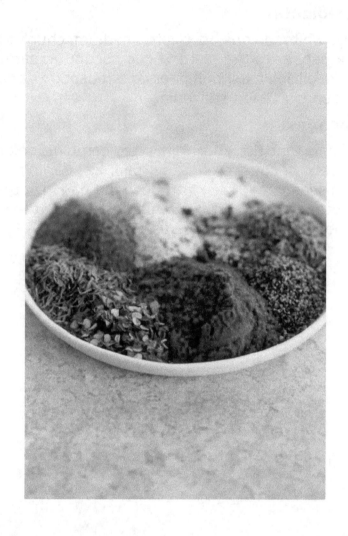

Green Beans Side Salad

Preparation Time: 10 minutes Cooking Time: 15 minutes Servings:

Ingredients

1-pint cherry tomatoes 1 pound green beans 2 tablespoons olive oil Salt and black pepper to the taste

Directions:

In a bowl, mix cherry tomatoes with green beans, olive oil, salt and pepper, toss, and transfer to a pan that fits your Air Fryer and cook at 400 ° F for 15 minutes. Divide between plates and serve as a side dish.

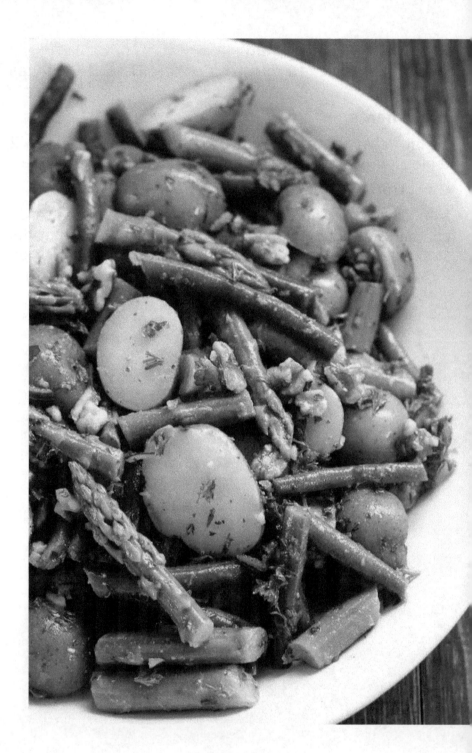

White Mushrooms Mix

Preparation Time: 10 minutes Cooking Time: 15 minutes
Servings:

Ingredients

Salt and black pepper to the taste 7 ounces snow peas 8 ounces white mushrooms, halved 1 yellow onion, cut into rings 2 tablespoons coconut aminos 1 teaspoon olive oil

Directions:

In a bowl, snow peas with mushrooms, onion, aminos, oil, salt and pepper, toss well, transfer to a pan that fits your Air Fryer, introduce in the fryer and cook at 350 °F for 15 minutes. Divide between plates and serve as a side dish

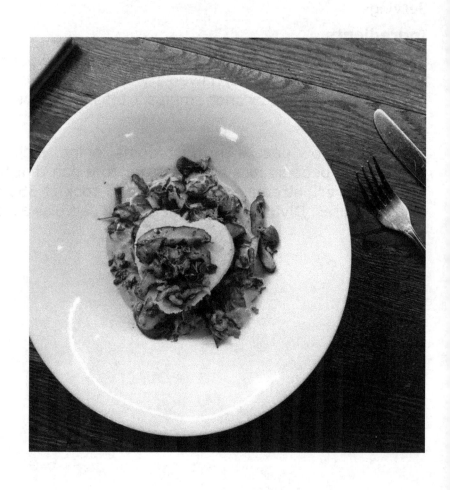

Mushrooms and Watercress Salad

Preparation time: 10 minutes Cooking time: 30 minutes
Servings: 3

Ingredients:

8 firm mushrooms, sliced 4 eggs, hard-boiled 1 bunch watercress 1 potato ½ medium-sized red onion 1 lb. string beans 1 medium-small cucumber ¾ cup Sour Cream Dressing ½ cup mayonnaise

Directions:

Peel and dice the potato, cook it in boiling salted water until it is tender, drain, and run cold water over it until it is cool. Put it in the refrigerator. Wash and trim the string beans, cut them in 1-inch pieces, and boil them in salted water until they are just tender—not a minute longer. Run cold water over them until they are cool and put them in the refrigerator. Wash the watercress, trim off the heavy stems, and cut in half any very large pieces. Quarter and thinly slice the red onion. Peel and coarsely chop the hard-boiled eggs. Peel the cucumber, halve it lengthwise, and slice it. Clean the mushrooms, trim off the stems, and slice them thinly. Toss all the vegetable ingredients together in a bowl. Blend Sour Cream Dressing I with the mayonnaise; pour the dressing over the salad and toss again until everything is evenly coated.

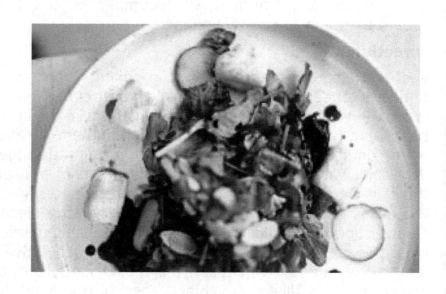

Lima Bean Salad

Preparation time: 10 minutes Cooking time: 40 minutes
Servings: 3

Ingredients:

2 cups dry lima beans, large ⅓ cup olive oil 1½ qts. water
¼ cup white wine vinegar salt fresh-ground black pepper

Directions:

Put the beans in a large pot with the water and 1
teaspoon salt, bring to a boil, then reduce the flame.
Simmer the beans gently for about 1 hour, or until they
are just tender. Drain them while they are still hot,
reserving the liquid. In a skillet, boil the bean liquid
vigorously for a few minutes until it is substantially
thickened. Measure out ⅔ cup of the thickened liquid into
a bowl. Add 1 tablespoon salt plus all of the other
ingredients to the warm liquid and whisk until well
blended and you have a smooth sauce. Pour the sauce
over the beans while they are still warm and mix them
up gently with a wooden spoon, being careful not to mash
them. Refrigerate for several hours. Before serving, stir
the salad again so that all the beans are well coated with
the dressing.

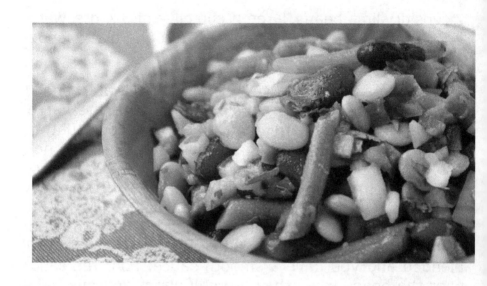

Exquisite Banana, Apple, and Coconut Curry

Servings: 6 Preparation time: 6 hours and 10 minutes

Ingredients:

1/2 cup of amaranth seeds 1 apple, cored and sliced 1 banana, sliced 1 1/2 cups of diced tomatoes 3 teaspoons of chopped parsley 1 green pepper, chopped 1 large white onion, peeled and diced 2 teaspoons of minced garlic 1 teaspoon of salt 1 teaspoon of ground cumin 2 1/2 tablespoons of curry powder 2 tablespoons of flour 2 bay leaves 1/2 cup of white wine 8 fluid ounce of coconut milk 1/2 cup of water

Directions:

Using a food processor place the apple, tomatoes, garlic and pulse it until it gets smooth but a little bit chunky. Add this mixture to a 6-quarts slow cooker and add the remaining ingredients. Stir until it mixes properly and cover the top. Plug in the slow cooker; adjust the cooking time to 6 hours and let it cook on the low heat setting or until it is cooked thoroughly. Add the seasoning and serve right away.

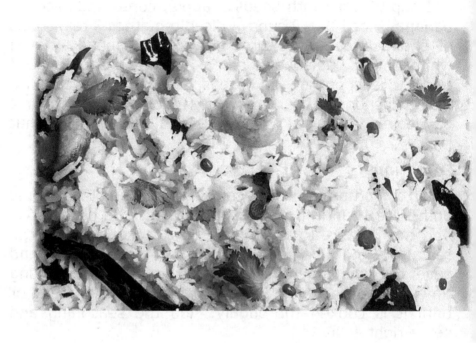

Delightful Coconut Vegetarian Curry

Servings: 6 Preparation time: 4 hours and 20 minutes

Ingredients:

5 medium-sized potatoes, peeled and cut into 1-inch cubes 1/4 cup of curry powder 2 tablespoons of flour 1 tablespoon of chili powder 1/2 teaspoon of red pepper flakes 1/2 teaspoon of cayenne pepper 1 large green bell pepper, cut into strips 1 large red bell pepper, cut into strips 2 tablespoons of onion soup mix 14-ounce of coconut cream, unsweetened 3 cups of vegetable broth 2 medium-sized carrots, peeled and cut into matchstick 1 cup of green peas 1/4 cup of chopped cilantro

Directions:

Take a 6-quarts slow cooker, grease it with a non-stick cooking spray and place the potatoes pieces in the bottom. Add the remaining ingredients except for the carrots, peas and cilantro. Stir properly and cover the top. Plug in the slow cooker; adjust the cooking time to 4 hours and let it cook on the low heat setting or until it cooks thoroughly. When the cooking time is over, add the carrots to the curry and continue cooking for 30 minutes. Then, add the peas and continue cooking for another 30 minutes or until the peas get tender. Garnish it with cilantro and serve.

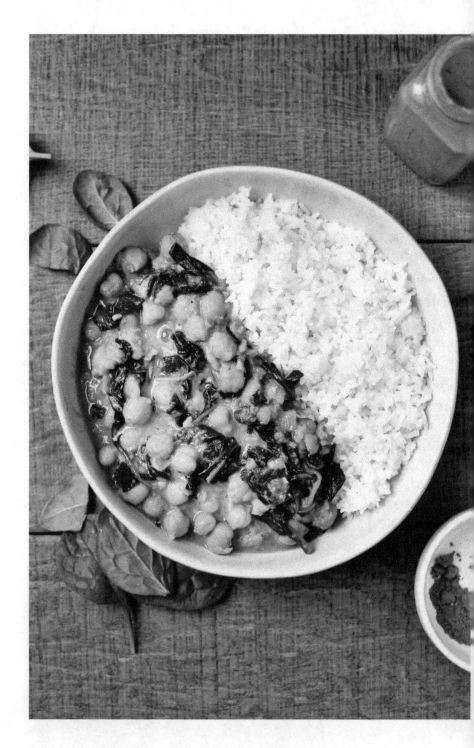

Creamy Sweet Potato & Coconut Curry

Servings: 6 Preparation time: 6 hours and 20 minutes

Ingredients:

2 pounds of sweet potatoes, peeled and chopped 1/2 pound of red cabbage, shredded 2 red chilies, seeded and sliced 2 medium-sized red bell peppers, cored and sliced 2 large white onions, peeled and sliced 1 1/2 teaspoon of minced garlic 1 teaspoon of grated ginger 1/2 teaspoon of salt 1 teaspoon of paprika 1/2 teaspoon of cayenne pepper 2 tablespoons of peanut butter 4 tablespoons of olive oil 12-ounce of tomato puree 14 fluid ounce of coconut milk 1/2 cup of chopped coriander

Directions:

Place a large non-stick skillet pan over an average heat, add 1 tablespoon of oil and let it heat. Then add the onion and cook for 10 minutes or until it gets soft. Add the garlic, ginger, salt, paprika, cayenne pepper and continue cooking for 2 minutes or until it starts producing fragrance. Transfer this mixture to a 6-quarts slow cooker, and reserve the pan. In the pan, add 1 tablespoon of oil and let it heat. Add the cabbage, red chili, bell pepper and cook it for 5 minutes. Then transfer this mixture to the slow cooker and reserve the pan. Add the remaining oil to the pan; the sweet potatoes in a single layer and cook it in 3 batches for 5 minutes or until it starts getting brown. Add the sweet potatoes to the slow cooker, along with tomato puree, coconut milk and stir properly. Cover the top, plug in the slow cooker; adjust the cooking time to 6 hours and let it cook on the low heat setting or until the sweet potatoes are tender. When done, add the seasoning and pour it in the peanut butter. Garnish it with coriander and serve.

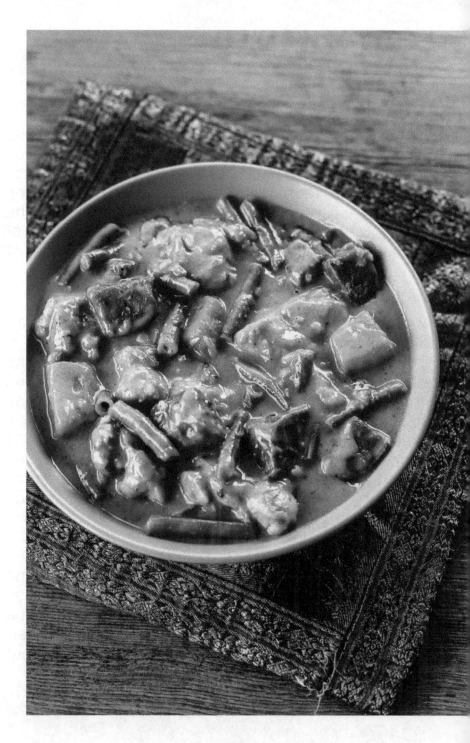

Black Bean Lime Dip

Preparation time: 5 minutes Cooking time: 6 minutes
Servings: 4

Ingredients:

15.5 ounces cooked black beans 1 teaspoon minced garlic ½ of a lime, juiced 1 inch of ginger, grated 1/3 teaspoon salt 1/3 teaspoon ground black pepper 1 tablespoon olive oil

Directions:

Take a frying pan, add oil and when hot, add garlic and ginger and cook for 1 minute until fragrant. Then add beans, splash with some water and fry for 3 minutes until hot. Season beans with salt and black pepper, drizzle with lime juice, then remove the pan from heat and mash the beans until smooth pasta comes together. Serve the dip with whole-grain breadsticks or vegetables.

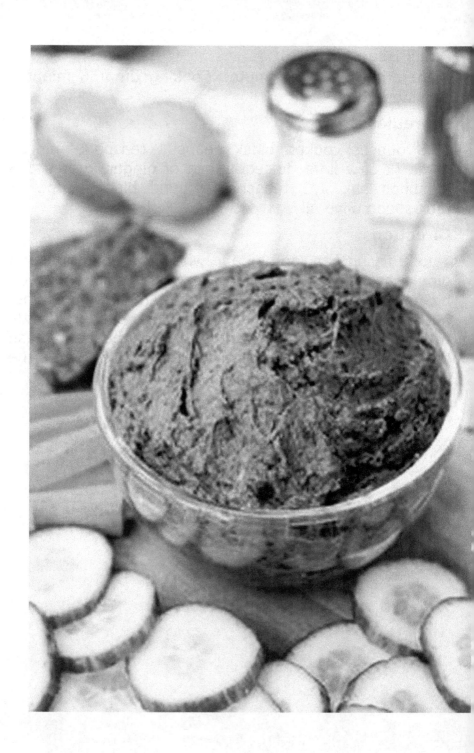

Zucchini Hummus

Preparation time: 5 minutes Cooking time: 0 minute Servings: 8

Ingredients:

1 cup diced zucchini 1/2 teaspoon sea salt 1 teaspoon minced garlic 2 teaspoons ground cumin 3 tablespoons lemon juice 1/3 cup tahini

Directions:

Place all the ingredients in a food processor and pulse for 2 minutes until smooth. Tip the hummus in a bowl, drizzle with oil and serve.

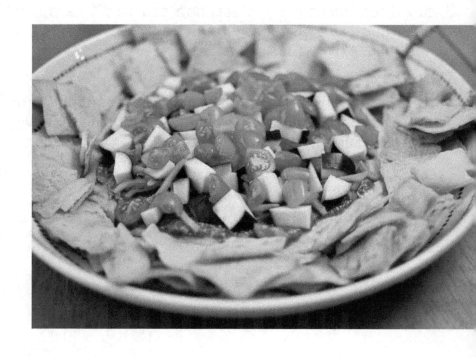

Carrot and Sweet Potato Fritters

Preparation time: 10 minutes Cooking time: 8 minutes Servings: 10

Ingredients:

1/3 cup quinoa flour 1½ cups shredded sweet potato 1 cup grated carrot 1/3 teaspoon ground black pepper 2/3 teaspoon salt 2 teaspoons curry powder 2 flax eggs 2 tablespoons coconut oil

Directions:

Place all the ingredients in a bowl, except for oil, stir well until combined and then shape the mixture into ten small patties Take a large pan, place it over medium-high heat, add oil and when it melts, add patties in it and cook for 3 minutes per side until browned. Serve straight

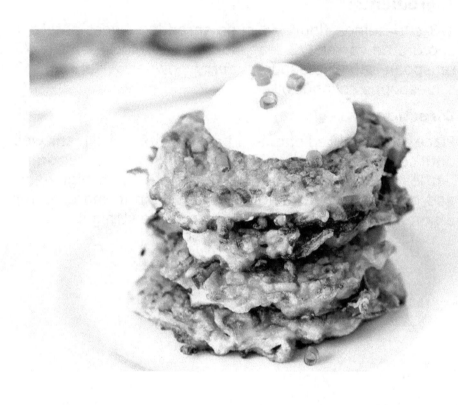

Tomato and Pesto Toast

Preparation time: 5 minutes Cooking time: 0 minute Servings: 4

Ingredients:

1 small tomato, sliced ¼ teaspoon ground black pepper 1 tablespoon vegan pesto 2 tablespoons hummus 1 slice of whole- grain bread, toasted Hemp seeds as needed for garnishing

Directions:

Spread hummus on one side of the toast, top with tomato slices and then drizzle with pesto. Sprinkle black pepper on the toast along with hemp seeds and then serve straight away

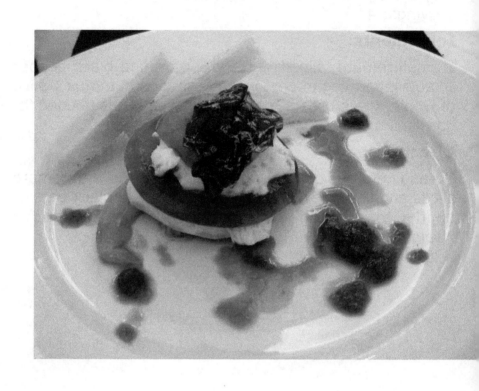

Apple and Honey Toast

Preparation time: 5 minutes Cooking time: 0 minute Servings: 4

Ingredients:

½ of a small apple, cored, sliced 1 slice of whole-grain bread, toasted 1 tablespoon honey 2 tablespoons hummus 1/8 teaspoon cinnamon

Directions:

Spread hummus on one side of the toast, top with apple slices and then drizzle with honey. Sprinkle cinnamon on it and then serve straight away.

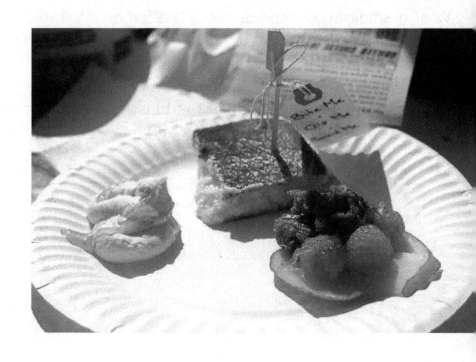

Zucchini Fritters

Preparation time: 10 minutes Cooking time: 6 minutes Servings: 12

Ingredients:

1/2 cup quinoa flour 3 1/2 cups shredded zucchini 1/2 cup chopped scallions 1/3 teaspoon ground black pepper 1 teaspoon salt 2 tablespoons coconut oil 2 flax eggs

Directions:

Squeeze moisture from the zucchini by wrapping it in a cheesecloth and then transfer it to a bowl. Add remaining ingredients, except for oil, stir until combined and then shape the mixture into twelve patties. Take a skillet pan, place it over medium-high heat, add oil and when hot, add patties and cook for 3 minutes per side until brown. Serve the patties with favorite vegan sauce.

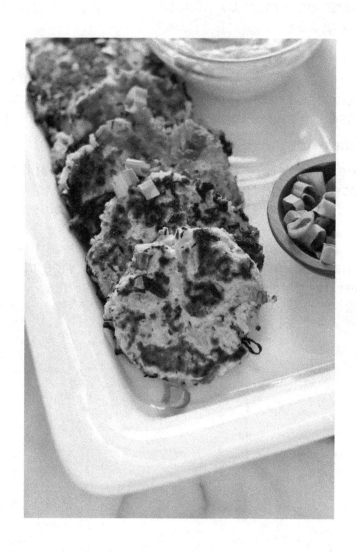

Rosemary Beet Chips

Preparation time: 10 minutes Cooking time: 20 minutes
Servings: 3

Ingredients:

3 large beets, scrubbed, thinly sliced 1/8 teaspoon
ground black pepper ¼ teaspoon of sea salt 3 sprigs of
rosemary, leaves chopped 4 tablespoons olive oil

Directions:

Spread beet slices in a single layer between two large
baking sheets, brush the slices with oil, then season with
spices and rosemary, toss until well coated, and bake for
20 minutes at 375 degrees F until crispy, turning halfway.
When done, let the chips cool for 10 minutes and then
serve.

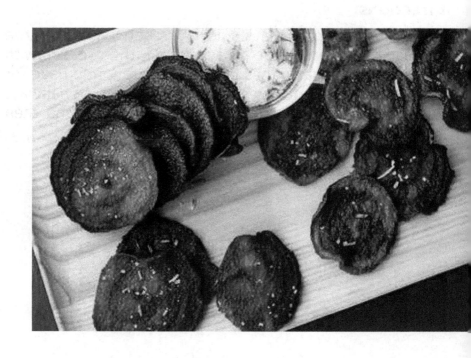

Spicy Roasted Chickpeas

Preparation time: 10 minutes Cooking time: 20 minutes Servings: 6

Ingredients:

30 ounces cooked chickpeas ½ teaspoon salt 2 teaspoons mustard powder ½ teaspoon cayenne pepper 2 tablespoons olive oil

Directions:

Place all the ingredients in a bowl and stir until well coated and then spread the chickpeas in an even layer on a baking sheet greased with oil. Bake the chickpeas for 20 minutes at 400 degrees F until golden brown and crispy and then serve straight away.

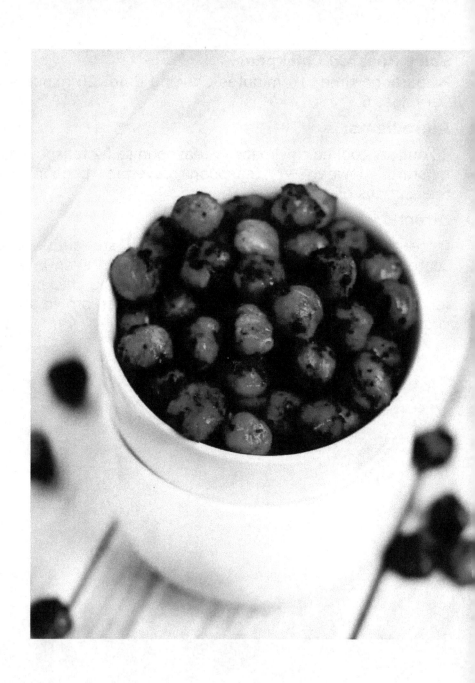

Red Salsa

Preparation time: 10 minutes Cooking time: 0 minute Servings: 8

Ingredients:

30 ounces diced fire-roasted tomatoes 4 tablespoons diced green chilies 1 medium jalapeño pepper, deseeded 1/2 cup chopped green onion 1 cup chopped cilantro 1 teaspoon minced garlic ½ teaspoon of sea salt 1 teaspoon ground cumin ¼ teaspoon stevia 3 tablespoons lime juice

Directions:

Place all the ingredients in a food processor and process for 2 minutes until smooth. Tip the salsa in a bowl, taste to adjust seasoning and then serve.

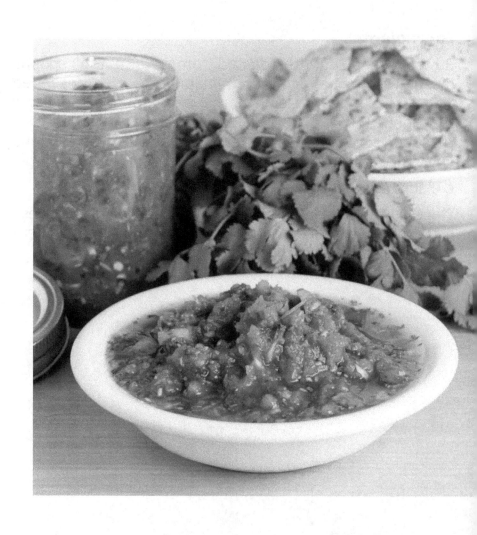